"What to Eat . . . What . . . for Longevity and Happiness"

"What to Eat . . . What . . . for Longevity and Happiness"

Herbal Foods Remedies

NATURAL SELF HEALTH
MANAGEMENT WITH SPICES,
VEGETABLES LEAVES, FRUITS

SHOBHRAJ KHATRI

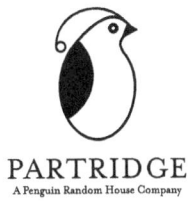

PARTRIDGE
A Penguin Random House Company

To order additional copies of this book, contact
Partridge India
000 800 10062 62
orders.india@partridgepublishing.com

www.partridgepublishing.com/india

Contents

Also by Author:
Shobhraj Khatri

"SWEET DREAMS" (SHORTS SHORT)

"LOVE AT LOGGERSHEAD" (-do-)

"MANAGERIAL EGO"(-do-)

"JEET YA HAAR'(HINDI)

"NATYA-SHOBHA(HINDI)

"CLIPPER" (MEGAZINE AS WRITER-EDITOR)

"WHAT TO EAT..AND..WHAT.. FOR LONGEVITY AND HAPPINESS" is a Health care Book written with concept of holistic health care achievable with the help of our rich herbal heritage.

The author's long time involvement with alternative &complementary therapies has resulted in the about day to day health problems with remedies from the kitchen and the plants in our own gardens.

He practices Naturopathy by interest and is actively for almost 3 decades in primary health care social services. He is of 71 years and well qualified BSC, CAIIB, GDC&A, and PG-Adv. Cooperative Banking, Journalism.

I have gone through the old copy of Book(Edition-2005) which is systemically formatted, the text moves from causes & symptoms of health problems with directions as how to prepare remedies at Home. These remedies, are totally harmless and non-invasive, can stem-out the ailments instead of developing into a full blown diseases.

(DR PRAKASH L. LULLA)BHMS,MD

About the Author

Main reasons for taking up "WHAT TO EAT.. AND... subject for longevity & happiness is UNHEALTHY FOOD HABITS & NEGATIVE LIFE STYLE HABITS. Human beings do not follow to eat nature's things available in our kitchen rakes, our backyards and close-by farms / forest without chemically treated. The information used in the Book based on survey conducted between the years 2002 and 2005 by author at places like Dhar, Jobat, Mumbai, Pune, Kolhapur, Khed, Baramati, Indore, Shirdi, Delhi, Haridwar, Amritsar, Ujjain Baroda(Varodara) and Rajkot.

Author extends his gratitude to the following person:

Dr Prakash L.Lulla BHMS,M.D.

Kanchan Godfrey Nathaniel (vegetables & leaves fruits-graphic)

Kavita Khatri (cover page-graphic) Village Panchyats

And Partridge publishing Group for providing Assistance in consolidating the ready script.

Chapter One

Falling Standard of Health-
Four Reasons

A small attempt on 'good health' management based on the various surveys and experiments conducted by the author at the cities and far-off villages.

Look the people storming and crowding the roadside eateries on Hand-carts, Cycles, small – cubical fast-food hotels and Mobile Dhaba to grab to eat 'grub' without realizing the 'end-result' by risking their PHYSICAL TEMPLE of Human body to roadside eating food habits..

The main reasons assigned to such Food-Habits are prompt availability of hot and sizzling and sumptuous food and at cheaper cost than well-maintained Air-conditioned or non A/C Hotels, which, still, remain out of the reach of the medium or low income families. On many occasions, even upper income individuals love to stand to eat just for the change and enjoy such 'junk-food' at nearly 'Mobile-eatery'.

Whether it is Mumbai's 'Vada-Pav'/ 'Pav-haji' or 'Bhel-Puri'; Delhi's 'Chhole-Badur' Or' Golgappe' ('pani-Puri' in Mumbai) or 'Dall-Pakwan' Or Kolkatta's 'Ras-Malai', hot 'kalebi' Dudh or 'Ras-Gulla' Or Indore's/ Ujjain's 'Batata-Poha', 'Daal-Pakodi', Alu-Tikiya or spicy 'Sev / 'sweet kachori; Or Ahmedabad's or Rajkot's or Vadodare's

Gujrati 'Daadheli' or "Masala-tea" in half-cleaned cups or food at holy-shrines like Haridwar, Mathura or Vanarasi.

A little serious thinking, recalls you to remember blowing and falling-dust, vehicles-emitting Pollutants, 'Ah.' chhi'.. 'chi'......sneezing and 'Cho...Khmu... Khmu... i.e....' coughing persons standing around cubical and passerby and also Cigaratte /Bidi ash blowing over the food you want to eat.

IS IT NOT HEALTH HAZARD, at none's risk and responsibility.......? Except at 'Your'. No health – authorities take any interest to save you from unhygienic 'junk' and take some sort of legal ACTION against 'Mobile – Hotels – runners' as the bribes control over the former.

The person, who likes to be servant of 'taste' of tongue, does not realize that they are simply falling themselves in the web of 'Diseases' Now, tell me, just... 'What do you eat...... for your good-health?'

'Do you not feel.. Uneasiness and fearful on your glutton eating habits..?' At this moment, even, for small – size illness / ailment, you run ultimately to the Doctor for consultation about Acidity, Obesity, Constipation, Headache, Skin-disorder, Slight hear-disorders and sleeplessness. In turn, the 'DOCTOR experiments with your God-gifted, 'Body-temple' by changing tablets and or injections.

So your 'pure' body now becomes medicated or call, intoxicated by the habit of the 'drugs'. Your 'Brain' stores such signals. Subsequently, it goes on asking from your body for more 'Medicines'.

This cycle leads to serious maladies to appear such as, Ulcer, Diabetes, Blood Pressure, Skin-ailments, Bones-disorders, Respiratory – defects, T.B., Cancer and weakness, on your Natural health which essentially in Supreme condition. A very crucial moment to control your fears of ailment and emotions of event of the consequences. Best way is to go on reducing the intake of medicines and reduce the food which you love most; but start to change, entirely, your food habits, increase the quantum of drinking water, particularly, warm water. Do meditation daily or Attend spiritual meeting of some popular Saints who do not teach you any religion or politics for forgetting the medication as the poisonous chemicals of the medicines deteriorate and misbalance body's symmetrical immune system.

It is very difficult to judge 'what is good or bad'

When you go to your doctor, 'you....know... what you ask him...?

'Yes right.....!

'What you should eat.....?

If you avoid the excess use of sugar, salt, spice and oil; do a few exercises or work on meditation / yoga even in normal course of life, no harm shall befall upon your health or Restoration from illness shall not take much time.

'Change is the Law of Nature'

By keeping this law in mind, change your food-habits from Non-vegetables to Vegetarian ways and further Change to boiled vegetables or cooked in very less oil and spices. Take care to eat less/ sugarless, salt less and oil less food for one or two days, initially, to adopt the practice.

Restrict your food by consuming slightly less so that your stomach can receive water intake comfortably and drink water after a gap of 10-15 minutes for fair-digestion in order to sleep, sit or walk without feeling the heaviness or drink during the course of meals. Avoid cold drink or tin – juices / food or even chilled water.

If you are under medication consult Your 'Doctor' for the Diets; but control slowly the medicines intake by reducing day by day, progressively.

Have a look at home-made food and its result on your health. I shall discuss the diseases and their modern treatment, supreme–health and retaining the values of the remedies grand-mother used to make from the natural fruits, leaves and spices on a many maladies diseases to have comfortable free and happy moments of life.

Chapter Two

Road Side Kiosk – Food

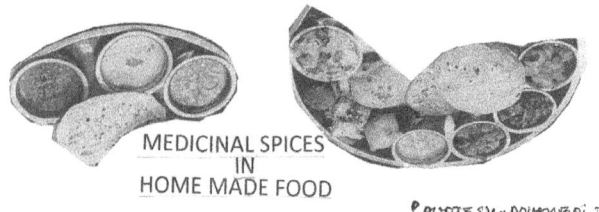

MEDICINAL SPICES
IN
HOME MADE FOOD

COURTESY - MUMBAI TIMES

Whenever, Some-one talk about food,' why do you forget', all 'eatable' substance, which are meant for eating, whether these are grown, produced or industrially made are meant for eating but under limit.

Nothing is cheap nowadays except the health of Your's and mine who run to the hotels road side kiosk for eating. The hoteliers, we are talking about, obtain cheap quality – impure oil/ ghee for cooking, Use stale vegetable - if none notices which are available at last minutes throw away prices, employ daily-wager, who may be suffering from some / other sickness out of hunger. Over and above, the hoteliers have to earn something for their families. They are helpless just because of unemployment. This is the crux of 'matter'.

Other side of 'truth' is that the health concerned authorities, for the sake of unearned money from such Hoteliers, issue a few licenses for official records instead of issuing to hotels. Whereas, the road-side kiosks are relieved persons as no Government/ Municipal office or Village-local authority would care for their stalls.

A clear scenario is None is bothered' about what the stall owners cook and how they cook! Ultimately, why should they bother and for whom? The servants of Government/ Municipal are mainly concerned for their monthly salaries which they get without any 'fuss' and 'threat-money' from the traders,

"What the authorities overlooked…? 'Forgot.. Their duties and responsibilities towards your health…!

Nobody is able to do anything. The Government has formulated many acts and laws; but the concerned official get scared to implement the rules just because of discontinuation of 'Pocket Salary'. If any official stands up to implement for unhygienic Road-side stalls. He faces transfer, instead.

The ordinary or medium class person cannot afford the heavy expenses of the super star air conditioned Hotels for the food, regularly, as these hotels recover high maintenance costs from the customers. So no other go. You walk down to Road-side stalls, Hand – carts, Riksha or Bicycles where food is cheap, without thinking about 'Purity' or Cleanliness' and risking your body. When will 'You'wake up from the somber and ring the bell for Your falling health!'

Even then you shall say, 'So what…'! I do not have time……!' let other people to see….'

Which people..?' You are pointing at.

Why other people bother when you fall sick after eating hot and sizzling street food?

You very well know that who is going to Big Hotels and or road-side stall to check the stuff they cook for the rich and poor, alike. You also know that why you are suffering from some sort of ailment by eating such 'crunchy' food. Any sickness is caused by eating the things which your mind does not want to give your body, but you forces your tongue to eat. 'What, then, if you want to suffer, knowingly?'

You do not – agree….. OK…..

You realize and accept 'Eating' causes any sort of ailment and you run to Doctor whether Private or Government.

All the troubles begin to take shape, now, 'Yes, now!'

'Doctor', in turn gives 4-5 tablets and or injection for the experiment sake. On next visit, 'Doctor' changes the medicines, if you are not relaxed. The medicines, whatever be the treatment, are poisonous chemicals. Your brain cells are amused by receiving the doses of the medicines. 'Okay – You want me to accept for your body',

The mind surrenders.

Such medicines are fast relievers. No sooner, you try to stop as you feel better, then these medicines start to harm some other parts of body.

Perhaps, 'Wake Up' call has not reached your internal ears.

Moreover, so far so good, many activities of some Doctors need your observations, particularly listing them out for you to note:

1. Many of Doctors in haste do not wish to wash hand, palms and fingers while handling cash with the patients. The currency notes might have changed many dirty hands. They start attending next sick person. The 'Unknown' germs may get passed on to other 'healthy'.

2. Inadvertently, many Doctors, not all, clean and dress the wounds of the ill persons, then, immediately, hand over the medicines with unwashed-hands explaining the dosages.

3. A few of them, with their scratching fingers touch the patients for pulse or painful part of the body with unwashed hands, lack of close wash basin or hand gloves.

4. Some of them, after operation, walk-out from the theatre without changing the apron and mouth-cloth used during operation and walk in passage or go in lift, coming in contact with other sick and 'healthy'.

Watch out and Safe-Guard yourself from such' minute' unhygienic trends you may get inflicted with the diseases instead of getting well. That too, temporarily, becoming well with the medicines, you stop using remaining tablets or other medicines and leave them on the refrigerator's top as good as forgotten.

After a few months, if you notice the same symptoms of the previous illness, without consulting any Doctor, use the medicines.

'Tell me, don't you do that exercise?' Then, how can the doctor help you in such pathetic conditions.

But you shall not stop or reduce eating 'Street..... Food'. You agree that Hotels or road side Kiosks do not cook food in clean and hygienic way. They use rotting vegetables available at cheap price, cheaper adulterated oil, heavy quantity of the spices, salt and heavy sugar for sweets, tinned juices or soups, dirty utensils, blowing of dust, emission of the vehicles, Biddies/Cigarettes ash from the lips / fingers of the workers and sneezing and coughing of the passerby and workers.

No precautions are also a reason of faltering HEALTH.

'Do you not feel that such eating – habits play with your precious life?'

Self – destruction risk by you and only you are responsible for harming your good health.

CONTEMINATED WATER

Even, you do not pay much attention about clean drinking water as you drink contaminated water without bothering about:

(a) From where water brought in?
(b) How is it brought? and
(c) In which pot is it kept?

'Water is boon to Man Kind.' Our 60% of body weight is water, even than water is needed for digestion, elimination of waste, regularization of body temperature and lubrication for joints and eyes. 1/3 of daily fluid intake through eatable or food and rest is water intake in any fluid form.

Potable water is chlorinated and cleaned with potassium permanganate solution. It is widely collected in clean-pots / vessels. However, cleanliness is not followed by street – food makers and even lots of Hoteliers use water from storage tanks remain un-cleaned for longer period of 10-12 month. Water becomes bacteria prone. Even bottled water is not safe from bacteria and higher sodium contents may cause diseases and blood pressure respectively.

A many persons drink cold-drinks, tinned fruit syrups/ juices for quenching the thirst; though they know chemically made plastic bottles containing soft drinks, syrups and juices have harmful chemicals like benzoic acid etc. as preservatives. By drinking such juices / aerated water, you are harming the body instead of gaining any fruitful quenching of thirst.

Similar way, you love to eat tin-foods which are packed in with various chemicals viz calcium nitrate, sodium bicarbonate, sodium benzoic and magnesium chloride work out to harm arteries to blood veins by 'slow poisoning'.

So Think your Self......

'What you want to eat....and .....What ......not... to eat....?'

MAINLY, THERE ARE FOUR REASONS OF FALLING HEALTH:

1 Unhygienic / junk food.
2 Uncleanness / Contaminated water.
3 Improper Sleep or Rest.
4 Irregular Exercises / No Exercise.

Chapter Three

Home Made Food

You may say 'eating something a little quantity do not harm or affect on good health management'.

Tell me…'Weather you have control on your tongue for sense of taste'.

Think… Right.. You do not have control…!

Then, start eating Home Made Food delicacies as you want to eat nutritious and sumptuous substances or you do not want to leave cervical hot drink bottle for the tongue tempting. Improve self control on even home food habits for your supreme health. Start reducing the quantity of wine / hot drink. if you can do away with it. Occasional feeling of drinking red wine is Fine.

There is a way out, take fresh curd with your night food for 15-20 days and observe the changes in you. When you take home made food, you are particular about cleanliness in cooking. Secondly, the nutritious food cooked deeply in oil, mixed with heavy spices and double salted is very much harmful in 'regular eating' habit. So keep control on such eating habits.

If you say... 'Nothing happens...!' 'I am perfectly well....'

May I ask you, then why do take tablets for 'Acidity,. sometimes?

Why do you suffer from 'headaches' or 'Weakness'?

Harassed by the thought of 'Disease'. Indian
Medical bulletin speaks about the 8 out 10 persons are webbed by some or other illness.

Reason is one... and... only one. That is 'Food' ... what you eat...!

Some families like to eat boiled vegetables without crowding of spices and without salt or less salt. Whereas many of families, which like hotel-type food, use for cooking a good quantity of oil or ghee or pure ghee, Red-chilly, double-salt-for getting iodine for memory. The former food-habit has its own health values as well as defects for not using a bit of spices which is useful in digestive system. The latter food-habit is total loss of Health.

Modern agriculture promoters or farmers want quick recovery of their investment for which they use the fertilizer / chemicals for faster growth of the vegetables, food-grains, fruits and plants for leafy substances. These fertilizers contain Sulphur chemicals which are no less than health hazard.

'What to do…?" is Big Question Mark.

You are not safe and secure in 'Food-eating-front'. But the world has to go on.

You have to be extra vigilant. Clean your vegetables in warm water and then use. Grinded spices like Kali Mirch (pepper), (Dalchini) Cinamon, (Badi ilachi) Cardamom, Cumin (Jeera), Kamal Patta (dry Leaf) are to be taken a little quantity mixed in vegetable while cooking in less oil and salt, during a day time main meals, is very healthy approach for the digestive system. However, remember excess use of such 'Masala'(spices) is rejected by the body loosing the advantages of the mineral qualities of 'Masala'.

The same way eating a pint of salt for obtaining Iodine for memory is healthy whereas excess use of salt causes high blood pressure and slow poison effect turns blood into water in blood veins. This is reason that why the sick persons have to take salt-less food for better recovery.

Normal person must take 3-4 mg of salt in whole-day, which is available from cooked vegetables (leafy) and fruits including Dry fruits. As such, one should not take extra salt to add on curd or salad. Besides main meals, you take breakfast and evening snacks and drink Four / Five cups of tea or coffee. For digestion of meals, you take sweets or syrup and increase the intake of calories and more calories. There is no full-stop.

Like salt which ignites slow-poisoning process, sugar eating in sweet, cold-drink, syrup juices and tea/coffee particularly, white sugar, damages teeth to kidney and harms blood veins. Avoid it and use less instead to save from obesity. You become fat by eating fatty oils which are adulterated with the help of cheaper industrial oil by unscrupulous manufacturers for earning more margin of income. It is very difficult to pure ground nut oils, mustard oil or soya oil without adding thinner oil.

How far can you save from illegal Health, Damagers/manufacturers, who are responsible for harming your good health as the obesity increases the chances of T.B, Diabetes, high blood pressure, Ulcer and Cancer besides \Arthritis.

Not scaring you as other diseases come along and dance around your body without any invitation as you have gladly accepted the fatness.

Finally, you land at 'Doctor's' or call up Doctor at your doorstep.

Doctor prescribes a few medicines as you want to get well fast. Allopathic medicines show the response fast to get you relief; but not without harming some other organs of the body since such medicines have poisonous chemicals which react quickly in liver, kidney and blood arteries. Even in Ayurvedic or Homeopathic medicines some or other harmful chemicals do exist.

I say that you can handle Self Health Management, if you control your food-habits, use Home-Made remedies from spices, the leaves, fruits, roots and vegetables and do exercises / meditation, even in small illness or in acute problem.

In a Maharashtra Government survey conducted in recent times in the interior forest in Adivasi family. The head of family inform the surveyor that no one has, in his family, fell sick for the last 40 years. They have never tasted salt, red Chilly, sugar or oil in their lives and they have not called up any doctor. Surveyor asked him that as what things they eat. The head said that eat raw fruits or vegetable. They do not take meat / mutton, Fish or egg. They drink cow's or Goat's milk without heating on the fire or boiling.

This message is they get nutritious elements, minerals and vitamins from water, raw milk, fruits, vegetable and leaves as it may be the reason for none felt sick in the last 40 years' period.

Think...think... and think... you eat oil, sugar, spices, salt and chemical milk. Your body has become a 'play-Toy' in the hands of the Doctor.

Start to control food habits with exercises /walking / swimming/ meditation.

Do tightly hold the 'health – thread' in your own hands.

Drink a lot of water till noon, reduce by night, change food habits and meditate for mind set to control the temptation of eating anything Eat when you are normal and drink water when you are indisposed or/at disease.

HEALING EFFECT OF LEAVES, VEGETABLES, FRUITS AND SPICES TO ROOT OUT THE ILLHEALTH PROBLEMS ARE ALWAYS NATURAL AND POSITIVE.

Below mentioned substances can keep you healthy and cheerful:

SPICES: Jeera'. 'Souff' 'Haldi', 'ilachi' Kali Mirch, Dalchini, Adrak, Hing, lavang, Madh, Rai, Dhaniya.

FRUITS: Ananasm Akhrot, Nimbu, Aamla, Khajoor, Santra, Triphala, Angoor, Anaar.

VEGETABLES: Pyaaz, lahsoon, Gajjar, Baigan Muli, Methi, karela

LEAVES:Tulsi, neem, isabgol, Til, Imli, Harad kokam Kadi Patta,

OTHERS: Dudh, Chhachh, Ghee, Madhoo and GulabPani,

Chapter Four

Diseases-Food Restrictions

Well... Well... I know that you shall ask me, 'What happens by eating anything of course eatable, that too digestible by human stomach machinery at any moment of time and what type of diseases occur, appear or stay or to say stick longer in the body'. 'Whether all the maladies can be cured with fruits, leaves and natural spices or herbs'

'Whether the better health results and longevity can be achieved by control on food and regular exercise'.

The answer of above health questions always 'yes'. If you have fallen sick, first of all, stop eating solid food or reduce considerably to be in good health in shorter period of time.

Drink warm water more and more. And also change food habits immediately.

If you are vegetarian and consume/take lots of spices, oil, salt, chilies with the food, cut it down to zero level and watch the recovery. In case of non- vegetarian, shift to vegetarian and boiled vegetables with less spices, salt, chilly, oil and sugar; because human machinery is not meant for digestion of flesh and meat.

'What do you say…?' 'Can't live without mutton…!' 'No problem…'

Change to sea food and then jump to the vegetarian way of food habit. You shall observe that your diseases substantially get subsided and your good health improves.

'Can you fast … for a day?' 'Very good' … Do it, at least 1/ 2 days in a week, eat boiled vegetables/fruits/dry fruits.

One or two cup of tea or coffee is always refreshing. However excess doses in a single day may cause digestive disorder and mental weakness in longer period as Temin or Coffin is poisonous chemical which weakens semen power and increases palpitation. Use 'Tulsi' leaves, if available, for tea as Liquid Therapy.

Whatever may be the disease? The reasons for the same are your food-habits, impurity of environment and unhygienic/un-cleaned ways of living style.

I mean to say 'prepare yourself for daily bath and better, if you can take cold water bath '. But during winter or sickness, warm water bath is healthy proposition.

Eat self made or Home Made food with less spices, salt, chilly and little quantity of oil.

Walk for longer distance or do running exercises or any other exercise daily for half an hour. Some simple exercises and yoga(s) are narrated the Book.

This way, you can keep diseases away and make yourself energized and cheerful so that you can attend your work and home smoothly and creatively. By not doing away with 'God of Taste', which invites you again and again to fall in 'food trap' and 'diseases' may send you their magnetic signals. Initially, human machinery tolerated your habits assuming you as new entrant in 'food-school'. But in a few years, you start showing permanent symptoms to a specific disease. Now, only you can consider as to on what stage you want to control your sickness.

'.....What...and how..?

Do.. an early Reconciliation, not with accounts; but with your food and taste habits.

Enlisting some of diseases which now coexist with humanity just like some pests. A few diseases, do not show up in this list, do indicate their existence:

DISEASES

1. Mental stress & Strain
2. Physical weakness or tiredness
3. Skin Skirmishes or Diseases

4. Obesity
5. Blood Pressure
6. Chest Pain
7. Cold-Cough
8. Vomiting and loose motions
9. Fever
10. Constipation – Piles and Fistula
11. Urinary or Kidney stone
12. Diabetes
13. Throat infection
14. Eye, nasal, ear disorders
15. Vein / blood Cholesterol
16. Kidney or liver disorders
17. Heart – diseases
18. Bones deformation disorders (Arthritis)
19. Ulcer
20. Cancer or T.B
21. Venereal diseases
22. Uterus disorders and
23. Combination of two or more diseases.

It is not over and all; but why should I waste the paper and more, preciously, your valuable time causing discomfort by the mention of names of the diseases.

Do not worry, in case of need, recollect the reasons for the changes in your good health and control your 'Eating Habits'.

Helplessly, you run to Doctor who experiment by changing medicines, injections doses for faster relief, temporarily. The chemical (s) in medicines may relief you from one segment of the body, you know, what may happen to other segment. Yes, damaging somewhere else in body, you spend a lot on 'testing' for temporary 'okay'; besides a valuable time. You taste / swallow harmful chemicals / element, logically. All times, a few medicines in certain cases, can't be 'one time only; but one has to continue to take whole life or longer period. Diabetic and high blood pressure patients are in the category. This is the precious time, when one has to control his/her anger, eating habit and to do regular exercises. It can certainly minimize damage control.

May I divert you from Human body to Animal body. Watch the routine of sick dog / cat or any other animal. Just observe and observe... sick cat / dog. It would not eat the food you fed till it become well. It would sit and sleep in sunshine. It would sit in open to breathe fresh air or roll in wet soil or drink a very little water.

Same manner, if you are slightly dispose off, stop eating food and drink cold or warm water, as the case may be, more and more. Do light exercise, if do not feel, do not exercise but take, slowly, deep breathing. Do meditation and concentrate on your disease and bring 'Well' vibrations within you by uttering 'I am all right'...I am

All right..' The mind and body response, positively.

You shall notice the changes within you when you attempt daily for keeping yourself in good health and shall feel new energies within you as you control 'affected segment' by mind control. Even in lying position, thinking process can do wonders as per 'Sun-Therapy'. Walking in sun shine for 10-15 minutes daily reduces obesity and rectifies blood circulation. Amongst Indian people, "Surya Namaskar" exercise is very much popular even in jet or rocket age. First of all take Moong water as far as food during disease is concerned, light food 'Rice-Dal' or Dal-chapati'. Add one fruit, boiled vegetables for second food without spices, oil and salt. Fasting is best remedy, if you can.

Taking Rest for 15-20 minutes after exercises would stimulate your hunger. Take milk when you are in good health and do not take alcohol and do not smoke when you are not well. Also do not eat mutton, meat or fish and white sugar. If you feel like taking sweet-thing, take 'Gudd' (Jiggery) Piece. Diabetics are forbidden.

Reduce medicine intake slowly and divert toward natural remedies for your ills of the body. Exercises and meditation can save you from eating tablets / Drugs.

'Good health management is happy life in 'Speed-Age'.

Chapter Five

Exercises and Meditation

"Prevention is better than Cure" is old saying but best suited to modern times. Human body means 'eating' and 'drink'. It has own 'self operating' system machinery, which is capable to fight the diseases, Virus and germs to correct your food – habits.

'Can't control the tongue of taste', you say.

'All right', you know that human body, digests or tolerates whatever you EAT according to timings, sends blood to veins and throws indigestive products out through urine and excreta. When the hurdles come in the way of natural process, you mind sends signals to body which indicates through symptoms of some or other disease for which we take medicines. If medicines / tonic can better your health, the doctors or their family members would have never become sick.

The scientific research have proved that the medicines are 'Slow poison' while okaying one part and start damaging some other parts of the body in a few years to come. Adopt natural process. Allow your body system to correct disease, within 1-2 days. Meanwhile, don't eat; but drink warm water, if you have fever. Drink butter – milk in case of stomach disorders. Chew small Ilachi (cardamom) and almond, you shall feel better in short time. Keep cool and lie down for a few moments taking deep breathing. Relax Or show to doctor, for emergency matters, who believes in prescribing lesser medicines; but allows you to reduce in short time. Keep drinking water as the researchers believe 'Water' is Nectar, the medicines are Not'.

'Then why not… keep yourself fit' with exercises or yoga (s) and meditation. Keep doing exercises for 20 minutes daily and do not stop once you start regularly for good-health management cause. You know there are three benefits of exercises /yoga:

(a) Smooth flow of blood in veins & arteries;
(b) Hunger stimulation;
(c) Physical refreshment and sleep.

Major benefit from the exercises and meditation is concentration for regulation of food habits, creativity and enthusiasm to excel in life and at work. Do such exercises which you find easy and convenient to your constitution. Of course, you might have done great exercises during your school / college. Even then, if you do 20/30 minutes exercises daily and fit you into cheerful mood, work and sleeping.

Exercises: A few of tips of exercises including Yoga (s) are narrated below:

1. Sit on mat on floor, hold soles of feet with palms with breathing out. Hold …try to hold for 4/5 minutes, tightly.

2. Keeping your legs a foot Apart with hands clung to body. Now slowly raise your hands and feet standing on the toes. Breathe in at the same time with 'raised' moment. Stand on the toes for a while holding your breathing. Then, slowly down hands and feet releasing 'breathe'. Do it at least 5 times.

3. Stand two feet apart and hands open up at 90 degrees of the body. Bend on the right leg forward till you can. Repeat with left leg. Remember to keep breath in and out with stomach inside. Do it at least 5 times.

4. For all age group, start walking with right leg put first forward at brisk pace and left hand forward. Keep breathe out. Walk for 10 minutes.

Yoga:

1. Do this Yoga exercises in open and pure airy space. Put a mat on ground, sit with crossed leg position and keep your head – neck – back bone in erect position. Close your eyes for a few seconds in a straight posture. First breathe in a normal way and feel the flow of breath. Now breaths in (inhaling) slowly and deeply expanding chest as you breathe and stomach in, Hold it there for a 15 seconds. Now breathe out (exhaling) slowly with stomach in hold for 15 seconds. Do it for 5 minutes or 10 exercises.

2. Calmly sit in crossed legs position. Breathe in and breathe out normally 3 times. Now close left nostril with left thumb. Inhale from right slowly to full extent and hold it and then exhale from left nostril. Repeat with right nostril closed.
    Do for 3/ 5 minutes.

3. After above Yoga, do the Relaxation, lie on your back touching the floor mat stretch both arms resting by your side, close your eyes, inhale and exhale normally. Start observing your own body is taut from little toe of foot to head upward.

Now slowly go on relaxing each smallest part of body up to your head. Now think of black hairs with closed eyes. Keep breathing out smoothly. Remain there in that position for 10 minutes. If you go into light sleep or trench, do not deny that sleep. It would make you stress free. It is called 'Corpse' or 'Savasan'

There is a many more Yoga for various types of diseases. But the above Yoga (s) is best suited to everyone in any age group for making you cool mentally; though physically you may be slightly tired with Enhanced vitality, concentration and serenity.

Sitting Posture of Meditation:

Meditation learning' through book will not pose any problem for you in understanding the method. Once learnt, the deeper you go, you can hold firmer grip on inner peace and Healthiest body and much healthier mind. You find many cults, sects or groups charge very heavy fees for teaching you 'meditation' for mind control. In your Interest, take 'interest' in proper learning the correct method of meditation.

Sit on mat / bed sheet after fresh up. Put right leg on left thigh and left leg on right thigh in crossed position. If you can't cross both legs, you can do with right leg on left thigh. Keep neck, shoulder and back-bone erect,

The palms on knees with first finger and thumb pressed together and other fingers facing down ward. Close your eyes and keep your head slightly higher than eye-level at round 200 to 350 upward. Breathe – in and breathe-out slowly. Start visualizing your each body parts from down to upwardly or to say counting from higher number say 100 to 1. Stay there in that exercises for 10-15 minutes and more. During initial days, it would be difficult to concentrate, but as the days go on, you will feel better control of mind. You can also keep your hands closely on your lap. Do it for 3 weeks, Say within, 'I feel better and better than before'. 'My pain has subsided'. 'I am feeling peaceful'.

After this exercises, keep your eyes fixed on pointed 'light-point' fixed it around 45 degrees from your eye level. Visualize any happy event or your 'god' who is almighty who made beautiful world. Or Visualize your far off relatives or friends. Do it regularly. In this routine, you are talking to self and universe / cosmos through your body Arial, which consists of seven stages. These stages / locations are controlled by twin brain hemispheres. The left hemisphere control the right side of the body and right control the left side of the body.

The right side brain receives any information and passes on to left side brain for confirmation and scrutiny. Your body gets in good health, if your both nostrils function rightly i.e. breathing both nostrils during meditation. The body Arial helps you for deeper concentration and mind set.

STAGES

During 1st stage of meditation you see 'red' (life energy) based at down spine.

2nd stage's symbol 'orange' at behind genital parts,

3rd Stage – you visualize 'yellow' – junction of energy (based at solar plexus).

4th Stage – at heart, the pulse of Universe – 'green'.

5th stage at throat represents divinity – 'blue'.

6th stage at between eyebrow 'Violet' – telepathy.

7th stage at back of head – 'white' – psychic sound.

Meditating at different frequencies can be mastered with long practice from 1st to sixth stage. Use meditation process in healing your disorders to be in good and sound health and live longer with simple food habits.

Chapter Six

Supreme Health... What...To... Eat... For Longevity!

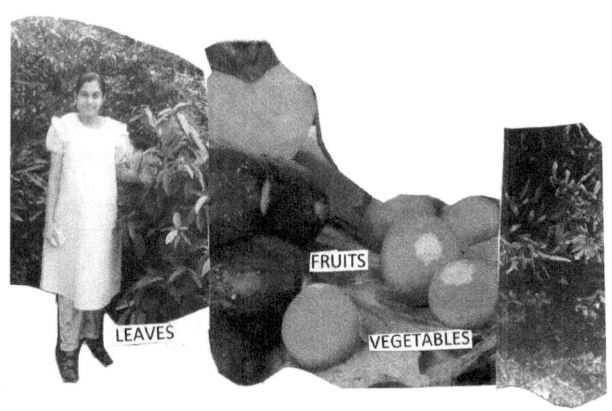

'Supreme soul leads to supreme health'

Meditation is one of the paths to purify your mind, pacify your emotions in the body and beget faith in 'God', who gives you courage to follow natural law and natural food' to gain supreme health for longevity.

'What... to... eat......?', is every normal and sick person asks, if he / she does not adhere to the controlled modes on food-habits and controlled emotions or feelings for peace of mind and positive thinking, continuous exercises, mainly walking/swimming/running or any other or yoga for fitness and relaxation. 'Meditation for reactivating the physical energy'.

'Yes... eat... whatever... suits your stamina... ', I mean, 'things' which are grown or made for eating. You can ... eat... things you like to eat which do not react on body, during your sickness or indisposed, internal / external body-system. Stop the use of meat-mutton, chicken, (the research excluded fish or eggs) which are not meant for human-digestion. Eat, under limited use of salt, sugar, spices and oil; though essential. Use Natural sources for green vegetable fruits and leaves. Use 'Tulsi' for fever & cough 'Pudina' for stomach ailments,

If adhere to, you can keep, yourself, healthy throughout the life.

(Here 'things' mean the vegetables, fruits, leaves, pulses and natural spices.)

What you need is 'simple balance diet 'containing 'Moong Dall'(pulses), Wheat 'Chapati', Buttermilk or curd (yoghurt), Starch – removed rice (Remove water from boiling rice) and boiled Or less oil – cooked vegetable(s).

At the beginning stages, you may not like / love the taste as your body is not attuned to such food. Try one / two meals in a week, initially, to facilitate in changing Food habits from spicy sugary and oily meals; which are deadly loaded with harmful elements. 'Vanaspati' or 'oil' is contaminated with other spurious chemicals and or industrial oil for the gains by the Manufactures.

You have not to change over you food – habits all of sudden as it will be risky and harmful to body. So design the change of 'likings' for Roadside eateries / Hotels food, slowly, to Home Made / self made food which may be cooked in less oil, salt and spices. Avoid non-vegetarian dishes. From this stage, changing to 'boiled food' can be easier.

But, the irony of the body is that salt, sugar and spices are essential elements which cannot be avoided / neglected in eating as it as useful as 'catalyst / agents' for the digestive-system and heat-energy. Best alternative is available to substitute with the fruits, vegetables & leaves. And also, a little bit of home-made spices is a must 'use' for the sake of medicinal qualities of the spices.

You know or may not know that how 'white sugar' is processed. It is mixed with quicklime, phosphates, phosphoric acid and animal bones for cleaning and whitening. Normal persons and Diabetic, alike, should keep the 'poisonous' substance away from their lives. Eat Honey or jiggery instead of 'dreadful sugar' for sweetening purposes, if at all you want to have the taste; but changing over to the fruits for the sugar required by the body shall save you from harmful results / effects.

Salt is also poisonous, medically proved by the researchers, as it contains sodium elements. It raises and varies the blood pressure in the arteries causing heart disorders and blockage/clogging of veins.

Similarly, oil increases fats in the body and blood veins leads to Obesity, heart and stomach ailments.

Water Therapy

In order of safeguard your normal good health, adopt 'water therapy' as a partner of your life. Take care to avoid plastic bottle water as it generates viruses from the plastic chemicals. Also discontinue drinking chilled water, in summer, which causes viral fever because of the difference in temperatures of the body and atmosphere. It is always healthier to drink more and plain water for normal persons and for sick, too.

Make a habit of 'water-exercise' as a 'routine' by drinking water without eating anything and without brushing at early hours of day as soon as you get up and have face muscle exercise. Join your palms together rub vigorously and rub the palms over your face 7 times praying to 'Almighty' to keep your health in good shape. You can start drinking a full glass or half glass, depending upon your initial intake of water and increase, then, quantity of water by half a glass after 10-15 days if you feel to increase, comfortably.

This 'water – therapy' cleans the internal system, increases resistance to the diseases and strengthen your physique. In an interval of two / three hours, till evening, keep drinking, when sun sets reduce the intake of water so that your 'sweet sleep' does not get disturbed because of Abdomen heaviness. Use warm water for sick persons suffering from Diabetes, Hypertension, Acidity, Indigestion, stomach disorders, Obesity, Urinary infections, Respiratory infections, T.B. and cancer. Normal persons remain well without pills and live healthy longer life.

An 'extra-ordinary' man only can take an 'ordinary food' as he is not tempted by 'Taste of the tongue'. Remember that you are also not an ordinary person and you can eat simple diet and plain water for 'Supreme Health Management'. May I continue with healing 'fruits'.

In Normal course, you should eat 1 or 2 fruits in a day which do not disturb the balance of basic Elements in the body. Pineapple, grapes, orange and pomegranate are the fruits good, even, for Diabetic with limit of one full or two half fruits.

At the time of two main meals, keep your stomach a little bit empty so that you can freely walk, sit or sleep comfortably and drink water after a gap of 5 / 10 minutes for smooth digestion and lighter body.

What Not To Eat-Controversy

'What... to...Eat..?'

Everyone asks: but none asks for "What... not...to... eat..' in normal course of life. Of course, when someone falls sick, in that case, you question the Doctor, 'What not to be eaten during sickness?'

A normal person should eat such a thing which does not harm the human body, or which does not react when he/ she is sick, for example Meat-mutton or flesh of animals is not meant for the suggestion of human machinery. Count down the things which do not suit your system or constitution and, then stop eating one by one with reduction in quantity. Do not stop/discontinue, food which you like most eating or drinking, all of sudden.

Many of reader would not agree with my experiments, observations, research or to say surveys. As some persons like a thing to eat and other may not. A very common confusion over the Eating habits in almost all the families. However, let up skip the controversial part and do some honest soul searching based on scientific researches and experiments.

Enlisted are things which should, in long run of life, be avoided:

1. Processed oil;
2. Excess of salt;
3. White sugar

4. Excess of spices in daily use;
5. Excess of red chilly;
6. Aerated water / ice creams;
7. Tinned syrups;
8. Excess of potatoes;
9. Deep fried snacks / vegetables;
10. Bottled water;
11. Excess of pickles;
12. Hot drinks / alcohol;
13. Smoking of any form / chewing tobacco;
14. Chocolates and sweet bakery items;
15. Excess of tea or coffee;
16. Proteins rich Pizza, cheese / paneer / butter;
17. Unhygienic street food.

It I say, do not eat said foods, your questions would be as to what other things are left out to eat. Not to worry, even if you eat less. But for good health, you have to bear with in life. The growing children need more vitamins, mineral, carbohydrates, proteins and what not. After 20-30 years of age, it does not affect much, even if you go on reducing the 'sensitive thing' which show negative and harmful result on human machinery. The relaxation to eat up to certain extent is permissible and under digestive limit leaving a corner for dissolution and water intake, in order to walk smoothly, to sit comfortably and to sleep peacefully.

Do not eat same food daily, but go on changing vegetables, fruits and spices system for intake of all values for human to have balanced things to eat. Out of various things, try to avoid as far possible 'four' white main culprits / enemies of 'human Energy; even for your children, namely;

1.   Fatty oils/ white oil
2.   White Sugar
3.   White Salt and
4.   White Rice

Adopt the habit of eating the vegetables cooked in very less oil or boiled vegetables with less spices. Adopt the fasting habits at least 1-2 days in a week. Drink your tea or coffee without sugar as it is taken frequently, not only you; but most of us, O my God. 'We forget to follow' is common reply. In a few weeks, you can manage and control your food habits which would guide as not to be tempted by other unwanted things in your lunch or dinner.

Follow 'water / liquid therapy' to ward off small time enemies of good health. It is a simple process. Have 6/7 glasses of water till after noon at an interval of 2/3 hours, but reduce quantity of water intake by late evening so that you can sleep comfortably.

Normally, you can drink milk, butter milk and water in addition to taking curd and slight pure. Take 3 times a week for a change and heat-energy.

'Extra Ordinary' man takes' ordinary and simple food' and don't fall into trap of taste.

Remember this message for longevity since you are not an ordinary person. Do not eat more than 2 type of fruit in a day otherwise it disturbs the balance of elements in the body. 'Annar' (pomegranate) and Angur (Grapes) fruits are suitable for all the age group. However Diabetic must take sour type one fruit in a day e.g. Narangi (Orange) and anar (pomegranate).

Importantly, during your two main meals, keep yourself slight hungry so that you do not face discomforts in walking, sitting, drinking water and sleeping. It is always suggestible to drink water 10 minutes after the meals.

I know that you know. Even then you carelessly behave towards food. Of course, oil, sugar and salt are essential for proper development of the body. Do you not get essential elements from natural fruits, spices, vegetable and leaves?

'Why run after the things, artificially, made from the "controversial" ingredients?'.

Iodine from salt, of course, is essential for memory power; whereas the latter is not beneficial when excess doses cause High blood pressure and kidney deteriorating effect due to sodium element, which is poison, too. Same way, sugar story can be written in full book. However a few lines are sufficient to bring out harmful contribution health.

Sugar is processed with lime, phosphate+ phosphoric acid are mixed and cleaned with animal bones. It dilutes semen and digestion power and increases cholesterol. Your body becomes 'abode' for guests like diabetes, teeth disorders, heart disease indigestion, skin – disease, joint pain and ulcer and cancer, too.

In order to digest sugar, body needs more calcium and potassium which misbalance the elements proportion and the germs, Sons-in-law of Health, dance around and in the human body.

'Getting scared… Wait for a while… ', you have yet to meet 'third enemy' i.e., oil. The fatty oils are processed with industrial oil (not eatable) and filtrated. Such oils harm bones/body formation, increase obesity and weaken eyesight. Ultimate destination is blood pressure, particularly, harms 'heart'. Similarly white rice is loaded with heavy dose of starch. Alcohol or smoking damages liver and lungs causing T.B. and ulcer. You can stop this habit by chewing ilachi (cardamom), Lawang (clove) and a piece of pepper.

In order to keep you in supreme health, do not forget to control eating habit, regular exercises and eating self made or home food.

Chapter Seven

Medicinal Spices Vegetables Leaves and Fruits

NATURE IS WONDER OF GOD.

The scientific research has established that the naturally grown substances have 'Hidden Nectar' which can heal 'diseases'. But one must be capable to extracts that essence to make human being well to remain fit and live longer.

In this chapter, I mention the medicinal qualities of the substances, category wise, whereas 'how to use them as 'home remedies' is also mentioned. Qualities of a few things or substances are narrated for benefit of the readers.

VEGETABLES:

Pyaaz (Onion): It has medicinal quality for stomach disorder People use in vegetable and chutney and also eat raw for stomach germs. Has pungent smell.

Lasoon (Garlic): It is very useful in high cholesterol, headaches, tooth-ache, ear-ache and stomach disorders.

'Garlic Therapy' for heart patients is very useful and gives better relief to control cholesterol level.

Cut into small chewable pieces of 3/4 garlic and ginger in equal proportion, half spoon apple cide

Vinegar with 8/9 drops of lemon juice to eat the concoction in early morning before breakfast as heart disease drug.

Gaajar (Carrot): Used for good eye-sight, ental and physical Strength, bones strengthening and palpitation.

Mulli (Radish): Used as digestive agent and for Urinary stone and eye disorders. Also good for jaundice.

Pudina (Mint): Used as medicine for indigestion and in chutney and vegetable for aromatic smell.

Baigan (Brinjal): It has iron element and useful in swelling and pain. Also reduces 'sweating'.

Cabbage and Betal Leaves: used for cancer medicine.

FRUITS:

These substances are, nowadays, grown fast with the use of chemicals. Before eating or to say for making juice, wash twice thoroughly to cleanse the chemicals and dust and or Wash in warm water or boil hard skin fruits.

Amrood (Guava): Highly natural source of vitamin C and potassium. Regulates BP and healthy skin.

Akhrot (walnut): It is dry fruit category. Useful on hair,& paralysis.

Annar (Pomegranate): It is blood purifier medicinal agent and used for digestive disorders, blood energizer fruit.

Aam (Mango): It is king of fruits. Used as natural sugar substitute And cleans blood by drinking syrup of raw mangoes.

Kela (Banana): Raw banana is used as vegetable & in urinary/stone Infections. Heals Dysentery and Constipation problems.

Khajoor (Date): Increases blood and provided sugar in the body. Reduces tiredness.

Tarbooj (water –melon): Soothes thirst and fever, used as medicine in Jaundice, burning sensation in Urine.

Kharbooj (cantaloupe): Coolant for mind body energy in summer and give Natural sugar.

Jamoon(berry): Very useful for diabetic patients to control sugar Level and dental-diseases.

Annanas (Pineapple): Soothes thirst, constipation and useful control Urinary infection & BP.

Amla(Herb): Very useful product in 'triphla' beneficial in Burning sensation in urine, giddiness, thirst and Motion / Constipation, also used in Hair Dye.

Papaya (Guava): Natural source of sugar. Used for digestion.

Badam (Almond): Natural source of protein. Used as medicine for jaundice, weak bones, memory and eye sight.

Apple: Natural source of oil. Used as medicine for hunger, Memory, blood and digestion as well a s in BP.

Narial (Coconut): Natural source of oil Used in cooking vegetable. Also used for worms & hair fall.

Santra (Orange): Natural source of mineral salt and vitamin 'C'. Used as medicine in jaundice, indigestion and eyes etching. Coolant in high BP and sugar controlling element.

LEAVES & ROOTS:

Ratanjot (leaves): It has a coolant effect. Used as medicine for eyes. kidney stone and urine disorders.

Imli (Tamarind): Sour taste. Used as digestive ingredient in cooking. Enhances vitality with sugar or jiggery.

Isabgol (Flea seed): White color skin (bhoosi) is used as medicine for constipation, acidity, acidity and indigestion problems.

Gulab (Rose Flower): The leaves kept in clean water useful in eyes disorders, Skin diseases, weakness and for weak heart.

Mehandi (Herb): Used for hair – dye.

Alsi (seed): Oil extract is used for joints pain, swollen wounds and Ointment with lime is used for burns.

Til (seed): Enhances strength and heat energy in the body. Used in Sweets. Its oil is good for joints – pain.

ChhuiMui(shy-plant): Herb, also known as Lajwanti (Shy on touch), used as Medicine in piles and bleeding. Also useful in uterus Bleeding & uterus disorders.

Beet root: It is used as in food coloring, good source of foliate vitamin Potassium, calcium and iron. Ample benefit in B.P., nerves Function and Anemia.

Tulsi (Basil): Pious herb worshipped, cleans environment, reduces fever, Mouth smell and skin disorders. Tulsi tea with ginger is Health tonic in case of cough and fever.

Shisham(wood): Medicinal agent for blood and skin disorders.

Neem(leaves): Medicinal use for worms and skin disorders. Oil extracted from Nimboli (seeds) is beneficial for backache and other joints -pain.

Harad(Herb): Medicinal use for eyes stomach disorders & hair dye.

Giloy (seed): Pungent taste herb used in high fever with 'ajwain'.

OTHER SUBSTANCES & MINERALS:

Lime: 'Choona' is used for white – wash. Used in 'paan' for digestion. It has medicinal effect on burns with coconut oil on swelling and pain with turmeric.

Soil: Extracted by digging 3 or 4 feet of wet place is used as dressing in fever and pain.

Butter Milk: If taken fresh, it has medicinal effect on sun stroke, heat, Piles and as digestive ingredient in cooking.

Milk: Top most health beneficial food substance for bones and Energetic health.

Curd: Dahi or Yoghurt, commonly known is a coolant for all. Blood purifier. It has medicinal effects on stomach, acne and weakness.

Ghee: Pure ghee is nutritious, energetic for mind and body. Medicinal use for skin diseases, snake poison, opium-poison.

Amla(Herb): Amla syrup is coolant in summer, memory enhancing, also used for hair dye, constipation and tooth & BP disorders.

Alum: Medicinal use in fever, teeth bleeding, red eyes and cleaning drinking water.

SPICES:

A proverb prevails in Indian Villages families 'NO LIFE WITHOUT SPICE' is true even in today modern Indian. The spices are used as appetizers, preservatives and medicinal agent. These substances lend color, pungent smell, taste and aroma to food, we eat. These products come in many varieties of shapes are sources of mineral and salt and help to curtail direct salt intake in the food. Nature provides protective Cell Structure to spices, vegetables and fruits.

Namak (Salt): Quality 'Black' and 'Sendha' is used for medicines. It is Always healthier to use 'Sendha' salt for cooking. It helps in food digestion, memory, bones formation and worms.

Mirch (Red Chilly): Its use as digestive agent and enhancing heat formation in the body.

Haldi (Turmeric): It has fairness increasing qualities besides healing effect on cancer, cold and throat infection. It has anti inflammatory effects on arthritis. Useful in cooking.

Adarak (Ginger: It acts in digestion in dried form and increases body-heat. Also act as medicinal agent for cold, cough, hunger and Bone pain and reduces blockage &mouth bacteria killer.

Dhaniya (Coriander): Used in cooking. Medicine for giddiness with Amla for headache, vomiting and burning sensation in urine.

Kali Mirch (Black Pepper): Medicinal use for disorders of stomach & gastric and throat infection.

Methi (Fenugreek): medicinal use for diabetes and constipation.

Dalchini (Cinnamon): Digestive agent and medicinal use in diabetes, stomach ache with katha and good effects in BP.

Hing (Asafetida): Medicinal use for indigestion, toothache, acidity and Gastric disorders.

Souf (Fennel): Good as medicine for indigestion, worms, weakness, Loose motion, ulcer (use with sugar). Its water preparation is healthy in normal time use.

Ajwain (Caraway): use as spice in cooking besides medicinal use for cold, cough, nose /ear pain, stomach disorders, increases Milk in nursing mother. (use with jeera and sugar)

Lawang (clove): Medicinal use on excess thirst, tooth-disorder, bad smell, Cough and uneasiness. People commonly eat in 'Paan' and Vegetables.

Jeera (Cumin seed): Medicinal use for mother's milk, digestion, gastric disorder and 'Coolant' for ulcer patients.

Ilachi (Cardamom): Medicinal use for urine disorders and excess thirst.

Jaiphal (Nutmeg): It has coolant effect is on stomach disorders and useful Ingredient in tinned or bottled milk.

Rae (Mustard): Medicinal use for digestion, pain and swelling. Also used for Regular menstrual cycle amongst women, sexual stimulant.

Multani Mithi: It contains drying effect on oily skin besides a coolant with Chandan (sandalwood) /khus(herb) application.

Now, I move to grand –mothers' prescribed'Remedies at own home–Natural foods as Medicines' from kitchen spices, vegetables and leaves from our own courtyards and fruits grown in nearby forms or forests.

Chapter Eight

Home Remedies- Natural Foods as Medicines

Day to day work, stress and strain, wrong food habits, fast lifestyle, pollution and global warming are overloading your body's defense causing maladies from cold to cancer.

You run to Doctor for emergency 'Wellness', but poisoning your health after intake of the medicines and or injections. At that moment, the prevention comes in handy. Wait for one or two days, if no emergency, when you are indisposed before going for any medicine as the body mechanism has its own immune process, disease fighting capabilities to ward off indisposition/

Illness and during that time you can start using Home Made Medicines till you show to Doctor.

Meanwhile, you can take precautionary measures on food –front to eat …this/that… or to have control unhealthy foods. Below is the CHART showing the ailments and the foods to Eat and foods not good for your earlier recovery from sickness/ illness:
(Without rule table)

Ailments	To Eat	Not to Eat
Ulcers	Dry fruits, Cold-Milk, sufficient water.	Oily and Spicy food in late night.
Urinary / Kidney stone	Raw banana, radish and barley water, beans.	Spinach & tomatoes seeds.
Headache / migraine cough cold	Ginger with peppermint, orange, sweet potatoes, guava, walnuts, plenty of water.	Chocolate, Cheese & Cigarettes, Alcohol and drugs
Indigestion, vomiting, thirst	Pudina & ilachi boiled water.	Deep Fried, oil, butter, spices, milk.
Pain-thigh & legs	Massaging with Pudina & Lime water	-do -
Perspiration	Massage soles & palms with essence of Baigan (Brinjol)	Tea / Coffee, spices
Swollen piles & wound	T ake hot payaz and haldi & apply / dress on the affected part for fast relief. Use pure ghee	No Alcohol & Mutton

Urine – burning sensation	(a) Cold milk mixed with water (b) Make paste of (onion) payaz and boil in water filter & drink water	Spices. Fried things
Ear – pain	Put drop of Lahsoon juice, mixed with suhaga	Sour fruits, Imli or chutney cold or hot things.
Tooth – ache	(a) Heat a piece of Lahsoon and Place it on tooth (b) Akhrot powder can be used for brushing	Sour, hot and cold thing
Jaundice	Raw Kela in milk/ sugarcane juice, Water and mulli leaves juice.	No oil, spices, fried food
(For diabetic, pomegranate juice only)	Pomegranate juice kept in metallic pot in night. Take with Jaggery next day.	-do-
Cough	(a) Take Ginger with honey. (b) Carrot juice with sugar and pepper (c) Powdered asafetida and turmeric & camphor mix in sugar melted in water and make small doses for 4/5 days, if cough persists	Fried, oily thing, butter milk, cold drinks

Physical disability	Foment hot water, eat grapes and sweet ripe banana or some other sweet fruits with black chilly	Avoid spices
Knife – Cut or Wound	Apply turmeric power and coconut oil. Drink lot of water.	No chilly till you are well
'Internal Swelling' only	Drink hot Milk mixed turmeric, Apply lime and Turmeric powder. paste	No water immediately
Worms (Common in children)	Give pineapple juice with honey at night and early morning for a week.	-do-
Blisters in mouth (Gurgle with turmeric water)	Eat curd and banana in morning, plenty of water ice creams	Salt no hot food No Chilly
Menstrual cycle - improper	Put powdered mustard in hot water and sit for comfortable time.	No Chilly-food
Diabetes (Check your blood sugar before and after 15/30 days using Home – Remedies)	(a) Walking for 20 Minutes (b) Drinking turmeric mixed with water for 2/3 days in a week and eat pineapple, Black berry & balanced diet two chappati rice and vegetable/ Dal	Totally avoid oil, non-Veg. food sweets, cold-drink, potatoes Do not be glutton.

	(c) Use (methi) Fenurgreek seed kept in water whole night for diabetes and joint – pain. (d) Drink cinnamon and bitter gourd juice 3 times a week 1/ 2 teaspoonfuls. (e) Control diet /'food' (f) Eat in morning powdered 'Aamala' with Jamoon-fruit seed (dried) with water. Use for a month. Go for blood test and see improvement.	
Joint bones pain and back ache	(a) Drink Milk (b) Massage of hot alasi/Till oil made by mixing Neem seeds and ginger.	
Hunger and thirsty (Caused by constipation and gastric accumulation)	(a) Drink plenty of water (b) Cold sweet milk (not for diabetic) (c) Eat ginger mixed with (rock salt) Sendha salt or cumin seeds with a piece of ginger/dry powdered ginger.	Non- veg food potatoes item, tur daal

Indigestion amongst children	(d) Boil a spoonful Sauf small green (Fennel) in water and filter. Give in morning – evening	Not to give bottled milk.
Excess Thirst	(a) Boil clove and cardamom in water and filter it in copper ware use for 3 /4 days. (a) Frequently sip water. No gulping.	Oil, excess salt and xhillies, no alcohol
Bleeding through nose	(a) Sit under water tape and drench your head (b) Take out juice of fresh leaves of coriander seeds and apple on forehead. Also apply sandalwood. (c) Drink cold milk.	No Hot food, salt, spices, sweets, no alcohol /tea/coffee.
Hiccough	(a) Drink or sip water slowly (b) Powder big cardamom seeds, sugar and chew the mixture or swallow with water.	Not to eat chily, salt and spices No alcohol

Intestine swelling	(a) Fast for a day. (b) Keep careway seeds (ajwain) in water for whole night and filter it in morning. Drink it 2/3 times in a day.	No food at all, No solid druit, no spices no oil or no pulses and no alcohol.
Nursing mother's milk (With this home remedy, mother can give milk to her infant even up to 2 years of age)	(a) Drink plenty of milk with pure ghee. (b) Add white Jeera (cumin) powder in hot milk and drink.	No pulses No spices No salt / chilly No Rice.
Paralysis	(a) Eat pomegranate and grapes frequently (b) Beet root (c) Eat cumin (raw) (d) Drink water of 'Shisham' (wood) soaked in water whole night (e) Mustard oil massage mixed with till oil + Neem /till oil (f) Eat 'till' and Jaggery.	No Salt, No chilly.
Dog bite	Make a paste of walnut powder, onion and salt in Honey and dress the part affected.	No Chilly No oil.

Bleeding gums / teeth	Dry the flower of pomegranate and make powder. Brush your teeth with powder for 15/20 days to see the result.	No salt No chilly or hot things No tea / coffee.
Dry / wet / cough	Dry the skin of pomegranate and powder it, mix salt, honey ginger dry powder make small tablets to eat for some days.	No Oil.
Eye – disorders	Boil juice of pomegranate in copper-ware and make it a thick paste to apply with clean – glass rod at night Paining eyes can also be cured with filtered orange juice / sour grape juice. Put 2 drops for relief.	No Salt No Chilly No Cold Drinks No non-veg. food No tea / coffee
Stomach – pain/ disorders	(a) Mix pepper and 'Sendha' Salt in pomegranate juicy seeds and take one time daily for 3 /4 days.	No Spices No Chilies No Oil Avoid food

	(b) For Twisting pain take walnut skin and rub on clean tile in water. Apple thick paste on nose. (c) A cup of tea with Tulsi, ginger and cumin also relieves pain. Drink for 14 days.	
Bleeding painful piles	(a) Keep (guava) Peru/ Jamphal leaves and skin in 500 ml water or less for a night and boil for thick solution in morning Drink filtered solution for 8 / 10 days (b) Eat boiled vegetables and drink butter-milk or pure ghee / cold milk	No alcohol No Coffee/tea no oil.
Bad-breath (and pain with bleeding at times)	(a) Gurgle with warm water kept for 10 minutes in mixed Asafetida, clove and rock salt or ordinary salt. (b) Chew Ilachi, rub ash of jamun wood mixed with sendha salt and a pepper.	No Coffee No Chilies No non-veg food No garlic food No onion No sugar / proteins Based dairy 'food'

	(c) Chew cardamom and lavang (clove) and sip water frequently. (d) If toothache only, make garlic piece hot on Pan/Tava and keep it on that tooth. Hold it for a few minutes or rub powdered walnut skin in case of bleeding and pain. (e) Eat pudina and tulsi for some days and keep mouth moist.	
White – hairs	(a) Eat almonds and walnut. (b) For hair cleaning use 'aritha' as shampoo. (c) Boil raw walnut skin, alum and cotton oil and apple on hair for blackness.	Do not use 'Shampoo' Do not use creamy chemical or substance No oil No Salt.
Stammering speech	Eat cinnamon, clove almost (no skin). Kesar, Silver foil (used in sweets covering) in honey for 15/20 days. See improvement and continue some more days.	No oil No Chilly No Sweets.

Itching, Acne (Skin-disorders)	(a) Boil 2 full lemon juice in coconut oil when it become thick and cool it for some minutes before applying to the affected part. (b) For face, boil a lemon in milk for thickening it, apply in night and clean / wash face with water.	No Salt No Chilly No Oil No alcohol No tea / coffee No non veg. food
Weak Memory	Drink 'Shahtoot Juice' With powdered almond in morning for 30 days with black pepper. Drinking almond oil 5/10 drops in milk sugar/ honey.	No oil No Chilly No alcohol.
Hard – hearing problem	Boil 'till' oil with essence of radish root and evaporate its water. When it become cool, put 2/3 drops in both the ears.	No sweet No Rice No Non Veg. Food No Oil
Perspiration in arms and legs	Massage Brinjal juice / essence and sip / drink warm water.	No tea / coffee N Oil No Spice
Smell of perspiration	Powder 'Seem' (Cotton silk tree) leaves / fruit and apple at arm-pits	-do-

Joint swelling (Arthritis)	Apply ice on swollen bone-joint front and back. Apple 'til' oil on green 'arandi' leave and make it hot, keep on it for some time Also use oak / Mudar plant leave. Boil fresh leave of mehandi plant in water. Filter it and mix with 'till' oil. Massage on the painful part.	No oil No Sugar No cold drink No alcohol
Boil / abscess	Boil 'Alsi' in water and reduce to make paste like put it in clean cloth and foment. It can also be used for 'arthritis' mentioned in above line	-do-
Itching and eczema	Apple juice of 'Genda' flower on that skin part.	
Fever	(a) Do fasting (b) Drink 'Moong' water (c) Make a syrup of dried ginger, Tulsi leaves, pepper by boiling in water. Drink 2 times. Eat grapes	No milk No oil No other spices No non-veg. food

| Disability, weakness or erectile dysfunction.

(Egg is also controversial food item as doctor confirm to eat egg as they consider it vegetarian whereas others consider as Non-Vegetarian | (a) Drink milk mixed with 'Fig' (Anjeer), dried ginger and Honey.
(b) Eat onion and Egg with honey.
(c) (For non-veg.) | No Smoking No Drinking No drugs / medicines No tea / Coffee No oil except Pure ghee |
|---|---|---|
| Excessive menstrual cycle | (a) Drink water with a pint of Alum or eat 'Pipal' leaves or "Babool" gum.
(b) Eat pure ghee in ripe Banana twice a day
(c) Apple / dress black thin soil on stomach | No Spice No tea / coffee No non-veg. food No oil |

The diseases and some of their treatments not mentioned herein this writing don't meant that theose do not exist.

Home Made remedies from vegetables, spices, fruits and leaves never produce any side effect. However, the persons, who are under treatment /medication may consult their Doctors for the restrictive use of natural- Herbal foods.

In any case, maintain an interval of 1/2 hours between the medicines (of allopathic, Ayurvedic or Homeopathic) and homemade remedies.

Author and the publishers of the Book do not assume any responsibilities on physical infliction continued even after the consumption of tried, tasted and positive result producing homemade remedies.

CHAPTER NINE

Longevity and Happiness

Human life, day by day is becoming hollow, just nothing in body and health because of faulty food-habits, polluted environment, irregular or no exercises, continuous use of poisonous medicines and no daily prayer or Meditation.

In order to safeguard and to save your precious life and to live longer and be happy in life for dear & near ones, Follow, a few useful tips for Good Self Health Management.

'Longevity Chart' is your Key to Happiness:

LONGEVITY CHART

REGULAR WALKING OR OTHER EXERCISES, YOGA AND MEDITATION PLUS PROPER REST/SLEEP.	CHANGE OF FOOD HABITS & REGULATE EATING HABITS But AVOID 4W EAT HOME FOOD & USE ONE SOUR FRUIT.
ATTEND REGULARLY SPIRITUAL OR RELIGIOUS MEETINGS FOR MENTAL PEACE SERENITY CHEERFULNESS AND HAPPINESS IN LIFE.	FASTING ONE DAY IN A WEEK OR FORTNIGHT AND FOLLOW DOCTOR'S ADVICE-MEDICATION

NOT TO EAT THINGS FORBIDDEN BY YOUR DOCTOR OR JUNK FOOD OR OVERNIGHT KEPT FOOD AND REDUCE DEPENDENCE ON MEDICATION SLOWLY AND NOT ABRUPTLY. SIMILAR WAY, REDUCE ALCOHOLS/ SMOKING.

DO SOME EXERCISES/ YOGA FOR CONCENTRATION &MEDITATION

REDUCE MEDICATION WITH DETERMINATION AND USE HERBAL FOODS. NATURALSOURCES

REGULAR EXERCISES / YOGA:

Whatever exercise / yoga, you are performing, continue to do the same regularly for the strength of the body besides endurance, alertness, flexibility of the muscles and creativity for better performances in your daily work at home and office. Any time is exercise – time except immediately after meals or in sickness. No counting of sleeping time.

'LIFE IS PRECIOUS GEM' given to you by 'GOD' and to maintain it in proper healthy condition by the food, exercises and yoga regularly even when you are bed ridden. You can rest one or two days out of a week. Besides your routine exercises, do 'Brisk walking' for 20 minutes and do not miss 'deep breathing' exercise for minimum 9/10 minutes.

PRANAYAMA YOGA:

Sit in comfort cross-legged erect pose and keep palms loosely on your lap. First of all, breathe out fully with stomach inside. Now, slowly, feel inflow of breathing-in keeping chest expanding to full. Hold there for a while till you can. In reversing the process, breathe out, very slowly, double the time emptying the lungs fully with stomach-inside. Slowly increase the number of 'deep breathing' in days to come.

MEDITATION AND REST:

Follow the 'meditation' process explained in chapter 'Five'. You can meditate in any position like sitting, lying down, standing and even walking(but a risky affair). Meditation' and Concentration' are two main 'gaining stages' for full benefits of the exercise. Here in this Chapter, I explain you a 'simple' form of meditation and mind control to treat yourself, first.

Sit cross legged on mat or bed sheet comfortably and keep your hands on bend knees. Close your eyes and breath out emptying the lungs with neck and back straight with eyes at 200-300 eye level. Feel that there is no weight of your body. After a few seconds, feel the morning sun shines around you, with closed eyes, visualize the sun is at forehead between the eyes. Hold the picture as long as you can. Praise the 'God' who created a such marvelous world to live in. Visualize air blowing, mountain height, river flowing. Concentrate on any Thing for longer time. It is a practice to control the mind. Do not get frustrated in the initial stage for concentration and visualization. In a few days of practice, you would feel, visualize and find light while meditating, resulting into a bliss, peace and might and fully relaxed.

REST AND SLEEP:

'Don't you need /want a little rest for a while'

I am not joking! A joke about lady whose husband was under my friend's treatment for stress and fatigue. She approached Doctor enquiring about his improvement. Doctor while handing over tablets said, 'he need long rest ... do... please... take these tablets ....'

'Sir, when should I give him....?'

'No....Madame...you need not give him...you take these pills.please...'

'Why...me....'!

'So that .. he can...'

Later o n, I came to know that Doctor had not slept for 2 days nor has any rest owing to over work.

Essence of Comment is rest needed when over strained, fatigue and tired after strenuous work pressure, either mentally or physically. It means body requires sleep which is supreme rest to restore its energy. However even after exercise, if you feel like sleeping, do not resist /stop yourself for 15/20 minutes of nap is healthy and pleasant. Or the change of activity also give you rest and relaxation.

A many Doctors / Westerners claim that the couple is totally relaxed after the sex –act which induces them to better rest, calmness and good sleep. In sex act, your body muscles do have various movements, just like exercises. Contrary to it, too much, sex damages the good health of the couple.

SPIRITUAL / RELIGIOUS MEETINGS:

Mind vagaries due to anger, lust, wealth, ego cause stress and tension resulting in diseases.

In such situations, attend the camp of well known Saints who can guide to achieve eternal peace, mental purity, self-control means and prosperity of health leads to wealth. Otherwise, start praying and worshipping your family "God" daily.

If you are contributing for the peace and control of mind, which render you to have control over your Food-habits to check you in becoming 'glutton' and to make you cheerful and happy. Develop a 'Smile' all the times to be more creative.

CHANGE OF FOOD HABITS AND REGULATE EATING HABITS:

Way to better health is slow process, if you do not have Determination and Will to change the food habits. However, the restriction of 'culprit' food is difficult.

So, cut down 'suspect' foods from your main meals and observe yourself for 2 weeks. Make water as your Best Friend in all circumstances. You can live without food, but not without water.

There is a living example of 94 years, the Saint Pahilaj Jani of Mehsana (Gujrat), India, who has not taken food and water for the last 74 years. The Doctors call it scientific 'Miracle'.

You are not such great saint, so seek water from healthy and clean source as there are number of sources available.

Keep the list of your 'like' foods, and 'dislike' foods and note their qualities. If your 'likes' foods list contains undesirable 'foods', slowly go on eliminating them and adopt to eat healthy and nutrition foods.

Let me, once again, pinpoint out that change to 'vegetarian food', if you are non-vegetarian. Change to boiled vegetables, if vegetarian. Curtail the quantity of the spices, salt. Sugar and Oil in your food, whether vegetarian or non vegetarian.

A 'balance diet' should reflect carbohydrates, proteins, vegetables, minerals and oils of nature standard nature; but in less proportion than hunger for such tempting recipes. Regulate and Eat your main meals daily at same time and breakfast 3 / 4 hours before main meals.

FASTING:

Fasting means avoiding all eatables and with water or no-water which will help the body machinery to cleanse out the sediments of 'poison' accumulation. It corrects the diseases of the body, which has natural instinct of a call for food appetite. So 'fasting' goes a long way of run in life, healthy life, in self controlling and strengthening will power for longevity, cheerfulness and happiness.

Start fasting for a day or two in week initially, but continue to drink water as change of food habits. Do not use alcohol at all during fasting or even no fasting, when you do not have carving for food.

DOCTOR'S ADVICE: A FINAL SAY-CONTROVERSIAL DECISION

If you are under medical treatment for any 'disease' or illness, adhere to the advice of doctor for your food and nourishment. Beware not to eat things which doctor has forbidden for your health as you might be in 'poisonous medication umbrella'. In long run, slowly, go on reducing medicines dependency.

IN A NUTSHELL

Eat simple food less than hunger, but at regular times, drink water at every interval of 2/3 hours till evening snacks, then reduce intake of water 3 hours before you dine at night, fast for a day on weekly basis, exercise and meditate daily,

Use homemade 'foods' and homemade remediate derived / concocted from natural herbs, spices, vegetables and leaves on illness you suffer for longer life, cheerfulness and happiness. Not to eat mutton and flesh of animals, not to eat spicy late in night ... not to drink milk, when fallen sick.

Eat pomegranate (anar) and grapes only in sickness... not to drink Alcohol... no to chew tobacco, not to smoke Bidies / Cigarettes ... not to eat food which does not suit your constitution and not to take medicines / drug, when slightly indisposed.

Finally, not to eat 'Street – Food' if not prepared in clean and hygienic ways. Observe the

Preparation of food and decide to eat.

In this book, note that I have narrated two different methods of 'meditation':

(a) With hands loosely on the lap and
(b) With hands with fingers clinched kept on the knees.

The energies, received from 'Cosmos' through the body 'Antenna' are circled around the body and stored energies so received from 'Cosmos' / 'Universe'.

Through the Body 'Antenna', while meditating with (a), the energies are released down to earth with total relaxation of the mind and body.

CONCLUSION:

Let me add a few Health Healing Tips to keep your health twinkling and glowing with home healing foods:

- Use red strawberries to soothe stomach ulcer.
- Eat carrots cooked in oil with increased anti-oxidants beta carotene soluble in fat.
- Figs have vitamin C for good bones at older age, but avoid raw figs cause irritation in mouth. It has medicinal effects on colon and cancer.
- You may call chilly are harmful. However, Not all the times, they are preventive medicines for blood clots leading to heart-attacks and stroke.
- Nutrient celery leaves contain calcium, iron, vitamin C, potassium and Beta- Caroline.
- Also Broccoli helps to off infection of lungs and arteries.

It is more effective through frozen herb having Beta-Caroline and Vitamin C heal skin ailments.

NUTRITION EXPERTS & SCIENTISTS WARNING:

Their advice to skip food items, as below, which may lead to complicating Health problems, harmful non healing elements and faulty lifestyle.

- Don't eat deep re-fried oil / ghee product/butter.
- Avoid too much of aerated drinks/Alcohol.
- Skip 4Ws- white Rice, white sugar, salt and Ghee.
- Keep off CURED and SMOKED meats of animals.

As last word, the suggestions in the Book on consumption of HOMEMADE REMEDIES

is being practiced since ages in the families all over world, tried on patients practically with positive results and benefits with improvement and surveyed by the Author at different places in India.

However, the writer and the Publishers do not assume the Responsibilities on physical inflictions or deficiencies continued with the patients even

After the use of healing foods / herbal foods as natural self –health management.

BIBLIOGRAPHY

1   INDIAN MEDICAL BULETIN
2   AMERICAN & BRITISH MEDICAL COUNCILS
3   PERSONAL SURVEY OF AUTHOR BETWEEN
    THE PERIOD 2001-2005